# Kidney Health Smoothie Guide:

# Nutrient-Packed Recipes for Well-Being

Desiree B. Hardin

# Table Of Contents

# Chapter 1

Introduction to Kidney Health

The kidneys are extraordinary organs that play a key part in sustaining our general health and well-being. Often neglected and undervalued, these bean-shaped powerhouses are important for human existence and demand our attention. In this chapter, we will dig into the importance of kidneys, study their various functions, and shed light on prevalent renal health disorders that impact millions of people worldwide.

1. Understanding the Importance of Kidneys

The kidneys are one of the most vital organs in the human body, serving as natural filters and regulators. Positioned on each side of the spine, right below the rib cage, the kidneys conduct a myriad of activities that are vital to maintaining internal equilibrium, known as homeostasis. Some of the important tasks of the kidneys include:

a. Filtration: The major function of the kidneys is to filter waste products, excess minerals, poisons, and other pollutants from the blood to generate urine. This procedure is crucial for removing toxic compounds from the body.

b. Fluid manage: The kidneys carefully manage the body's fluid levels, ensuring that we do not get dehydrated or retain excess water. They alter the quantity of water expelled in urine dependent on the body's demands.

c. Blood Pressure Regulation: The kidneys assist control blood pressure by producing hormones that alter the constriction or dilation of blood vessels. Proper blood pressure is vital for cardiovascular health.

d. Acid-Base Balance: Kidneys manage the body's acid-base balance, preventing the blood from becoming overly acidic or too alkaline. This equilibrium is crucial for different metabolic processes to work efficiently.

g. Red Blood Cell Production: The kidneys create a hormone known as erythropoietin, which encourages the bone marrow to generate red blood cells. These cells deliver oxygen throughout the body.

f. Vitamin D Activation: Kidneys play a role in activating vitamin D, which is crucial for calcium absorption and bone health.

2. How the Kidneys Function

Understanding the complicated workings of the kidneys helps us grasp their complexity and recognize the value of preserving their health. The fundamental process of kidney function may be stated in the following steps:

a. Filtration: Blood enters the kidneys via tiny filtering units called nephrons. Each kidney has millions of nephrons, which consist of a glomerulus and a tubule. The glomerulus filters the blood, enabling waste materials and surplus chemicals to flow into the tubule.

b. Reabsorption: As the filtered blood passes through the tubule, important chemicals including water, glucose, and electrolytes are reabsorbed back into the circulation. This procedure ensures that important nutrients are preserved and not expelled in urine.

c. Secretion: In addition to filtration, the kidneys also release some waste materials and excess chemicals straight into the tubules, further eliminating them from the circulation.

d. Urine Formation: After passing through the tubules, the filtered and processed blood exits the kidneys, while the leftover waste and surplus chemicals create urine. The urine subsequently flows through the ureters and is held in the bladder until evacuation.

# 3. Common Kidney Health Issues

Despite their vital role, the kidneys are prone to many health conditions that may compromise their function. Some of the prevalent renal health disorders include:

a. Chronic Kidney Disease (CKD): This disease refers to the steady decline of kidney function over time. It may be caused by many conditions such as diabetes, hypertension, autoimmune illnesses, and hereditary problems.

a. Kidney Stones: Kidney stones are hard mineral and salt deposits that can develop in the kidneys, causing severe pain and suffering. They may be a consequence of poor hydration or specific food choices.

c. Urinary system Infections (UTIs): UTIs arise when bacteria enter the urinary system, leading to irritation and infection. If left untreated, UTIs may spread to the kidneys and create more serious consequences.

d. Polycystic Kidney Disease (PKD): PKD is a hereditary illness characterized by the creation of fluid-filled cysts in the kidneys, which may lead to kidney enlargement and impair function.

g. Kidney Infections (Pyelonephritis): Pyelonephritis is a serious kidney infection that may occur from untreated UTIs. It needs quick medical intervention to avoid additional damage to the kidneys.

In conclusion, the kidneys are crucial organs that conduct various critical processes required for sustaining general health. Understanding their importance, the intricacy of their functioning, and frequent kidney health disorders is the first step towards encouraging renal well-being and minimizing future consequences. This book will further investigate how we may promote kidney health via correct diet, including the introduction of kidney-friendly smoothies into our everyday life.

# Chapter 2

Nutrition and Kidney Health

Proper diet has a key role in sustaining kidney health and general well-being. What we consume immediately effects our kidneys' function and may either support or strain these critical organs. In this chapter, we will discuss the role of nutrition in kidney health, identify critical nutrients that support normal kidney function, and highlight foods that should be avoided to preserve these vital organs.

1. The Role of Diet in Maintaining Kidney Health

A well-balanced diet is vital for maintaining renal health and minimizing kidney-related problems. The appropriate nutrition may help:

a. Manage Blood Pressure: High blood pressure (hypertension) is a substantial risk factor for kidney injury. Eating a balanced diet that includes plenty of fruits, vegetables, whole grains, and low-fat dairy products can help keep your blood pressure in check.

a. Control Blood Sugar: Individuals with diabetes are at a higher risk of developing kidney issues. Controlling blood sugar with a balanced diet is vital in preserving the kidneys from injury.

c. Maintain a Healthy Weight: Obesity and overweight may strain the kidneys and raise the risk of renal disease. A balanced diet may assist maintain a healthy weight and lower this risk.

d. Prevent Kidney Stones: Certain eating habits might lead to the production of kidney stones. A kidney-friendly diet may help avoid their growth.

a. Reduce Protein Waste: The breakdown of protein produces waste that the kidneys must filter. A well-regulated protein intake may lessen the stress on the kidneys.

f. Promote General Health: A balanced diet that matches the body's nutritional demands improves general health, which in turn helps kidney function.

2. Nutrients Essential for Kidney Function

Several nutrients are especially crucial for sustaining renal function and overall kidney health. These include:

a. Potassium: Potassium is necessary for neuron function, muscle control, and heart health. However, persons with renal difficulties may need to restrict potassium consumption, since the kidneys may struggle to eliminate excess potassium from the blood.

c. Phosphorus: Healthy kidneys assist regulate phosphorus levels in the body. When kidneys are impaired, phosphorus levels may increase, leading to bone and heart issues.

c. salt: Excessive salt consumption may lead to high blood pressure and fluid retention, increasing strain on the kidneys. Reducing salt intake is vital for renal health.

d. Fluids: Staying sufficiently hydrated is vital for kidney function. Proper water helps the kidneys clear away waste and poisons properly.

a. Protein: While protein is required for tissue repair and development, excessive protein consumption can stress the kidneys. Finding the appropriate balance is critical for kidney health.

f. Antioxidants: Antioxidants, such as vitamins C and E, help protect the kidneys from oxidative stress and inflammation.

3. Foods to Avoid for Kidney Health

Certain meals may be especially damaging to those with renal disorders or those at risk of kidney problems. It is essential to try to reduce or steer clear of:

a. High-Potassium Foods: Bananas, oranges, potatoes, tomatoes, and avocados are examples of high-potassium foods that may need to be limited in a kidney-friendly diet.

b. rich-Phosphorus Foods: Dairy products, nuts, seeds, and some whole grains are rich in phosphorus and should be reduced for persons with poor kidney function.

c. Sodium-Rich meals: Processed meals, canned soups, and salty snacks may considerably add to sodium consumption, which should be reduced for kidney health.

d. Excessive Protein: Reducing the consumption of red meat, poultry, and processed meats will help regulate protein waste and alleviate the kidneys' strain.

a. Sugary Foods and Beverages: High sugar consumption can worsen diabetes and contribute to kidney damage.

f. Alcohol and Caffeine: Both alcohol and caffeine may dehydrate the body, placing extra pressure on the kidneys.

In conclusion, diet plays a key role in promoting kidney health and reducing renal-related problems. A balanced diet that emphasizes vital nutrients and avoids hazardous foods might help people maintain optimum kidney function and overall well-being. Understanding the relevance of nutrition in kidney health creates the groundwork for the kidney-friendly smoothie recipes and dietary advice that will be discussed in the later chapters of this book.

# Chapter 3

The Power of Smoothies for Kidney Health

Smoothies have developed as a popular and effective strategy to improve kidney health and general well-being. These nutrient-packed drinks provide a wealth of benefits that may pleasantly influence the kidneys and contribute to a balanced diet. In this chapter, we will discuss why smoothies are excellent for kidneys, the benefits of including them in your diet, and crucial strategies for producing kidney-friendly smoothies that feed and preserve these critical organs.

1. Why Smoothies are Beneficial for Kidneys

Smoothies provide a quick and pleasant manner of providing critical nutrients to the body, making them especially helpful for kidney health. Here are some reasons why smoothies are helpful for kidneys:

a. Hydration Support: Adequate hydration is critical for kidney function, and smoothies offer an easy and delicious method to remain hydrated, particularly for people who struggle to drink enough water throughout the day.

b.    Nutrient    Density:    Kidney-friendly smoothies may be filled with a range of nutrient-dense components such as fruits, vegetables, and seeds. These substances contain vitamins, minerals, antioxidants, and other vital components that improve kidney function.

c. Controlled Portions: Smoothies allow for exact portion control, making it simpler to manage potassium, phosphorus, sodium, and protein consumption, which is critical for persons with renal disorders.

d. Blending for Easy Digestion: The blending process breaks down fibrous components of fruits and vegetables, making them simpler to digest and absorb, thereby minimizing possible gastrointestinal pressure on the kidneys.

g. practical Meal Replacement: Smoothies may serve as practical meal replacements, particularly for people with hectic schedules or diminished appetites. They guarantee that critical nutrients are still delivered to promote kidney health.

f. Natural Detoxification: Certain smoothie components, such as leafy greens and citrus fruits, provide natural detoxifying capabilities that improve the body's entire cleaning process, including kidney function.

2. Advantages of Incorporating Smoothies into Your Diet

Introducing kidney-friendly smoothies into your diet may provide various benefits that lead to enhanced kidney health and overall well-being. Some advantages of adding smoothies to your everyday routine include:

a. Enhanced Nutrient Intake: Smoothies allow for a diversified assortment of fruits, vegetables, and superfoods to be blended, increasing nutrient intake and delivering a wide array of health advantages.

c. Improved Digestion: Blending fruits and vegetables makes them simpler to digest, leading to greater absorption of key nutrients.

c. Weight Management: Smoothies may be customized to help weight management efforts, which is vital for minimizing pressure on the kidneys.

d. Boosted Energy Levels: The combination of nutrient-dense components may give a natural energy boost, improving overall vitality and well-being.

e. Supports Blood Pressure Regulation: Kidney-friendly smoothies may include nutrients rich in potassium and antioxidants, which help to improve blood pressure management.

f. Variety and Creativity: The diversity of smoothies allows for creativity in the kitchen, making it pleasurable to explore new taste combinations and uncover tasty kidney-friendly dishes.

3. Tips for Preparing Kidney-Friendly Smoothies

Creating kidney-friendly smoothies demands deliberate ingredient selection and preparation procedures. Here are some crucial guidelines to guarantee your smoothies are kidney-friendly and nutritious:

a. Monitor Potassium and Phosphorus: Choose low-potassium fruits and vegetables, and avoid high-phosphorus items to preserve kidney health.

b. Mindful Protein Choices: Opt for low-phosphorus protein sources like almond milk, hemp seeds, or pea protein, while being careful with animal-based proteins.

b. Manage Fluid Intake: Factor in the fluid content of your smoothies to ensure you are not overdosing on fluids, especially if you are on fluid restrictions.

d. Herbal Additions: Consider integrating kidney-supportive herbs like parsley or dandelion greens into your smoothies.

a. Avoid High-Sugar Ingredients: Limit added sugars and go for naturally sweet foods like berries or apples.

f. Adjust to Personal Preferences: Tailor smoothie recipes to fit your taste preferences and dietary constraints while keeping them kidney-friendly.

In conclusion, the efficacy of smoothies for kidney health rests in their capacity to give a nutrient-dense and simple method to assist the kidneys. By knowing the benefits of smoothies, and the advantages they provide, and using crucial guidelines for preparation, people may harness the potential of smoothies as a helpful tool in supporting renal health and general well-being. The next chapters will dig into kidney-friendly smoothie recipes that contain healthy ingredients, intended to optimize their advantages for renal function

# Chapter 4

Kidney-Friendly Ingredients for Smoothies

To produce kidney-friendly smoothies that promote good kidney function, a careful selection of components is required. In this chapter, we will cover three essential types of kidney-friendly nutrients: low-potassium fruits and vegetables, high-quality proteins, and hydration-boosting substances. By integrating these nutrients into your smoothies, you can guarantee they give food while improving the well-being of your kidneys.

1. Low-Potassium Fruits and Vegetables

Maintaining healthy potassium levels is critical for persons with renal difficulties. While potassium is needed for several body activities, excessive potassium may put pressure on the kidneys. Here are some low-potassium fruits and vegetables that are great for kidney-friendly smoothies:

a. Berries: Strawberries, blueberries, raspberries, and blackberries are rich in antioxidants and low in potassium, making them good options for kidney health.

b. Apples: Apples are a tasty and low-potassium fruit that provides natural sweetness to your smoothies without overloading your kidneys.

c. Cucumber: Cucumbers are hydrating and low in potassium, offering a refreshing addition to your smoothies.

d. Pineapple: Pineapple is a tropical fruit that provides a tropical flavor to your smoothies while being relatively low in potassium.

a. Peaches: Peaches are not just low in potassium but also a wonderful source of vitamins and minerals to boost overall wellness.

f. Carrots: Carrots give a beautiful color and a mild natural sweetness to your smoothies without adding excessive potassium.

## 2. High-Quality Proteins for Kidney Health

Incorporating the correct proteins into your kidney-friendly smoothies is crucial for tissue healing and general kidney health. Opt for proteins that are low in phosphorus to decrease pressure on the kidneys. Here are some high-quality protein sources to consider:

a. Hemp Seeds: Hemp seeds are a good plant-based protein source, low in phosphorus, and high in omega-3 fatty acids.

b. Chia Seeds: Chia seeds are protein-packed and include soluble fiber, delivering a nutritional boost to your smoothies.

c. Almond Milk: Unsweetened almond milk is a low-phosphorus alternative to dairy milk, providing smoothness to your smoothies.

d. Flaxseed: Flaxseed is an excellent source of protein, fiber, and healthy fats, all of which contribute to kidney function.

f. Greek Yogurt (in moderation): For those who can stomach dairy, Greek yogurt is a protein-rich choice. Choose low-fat or non-fat variants and eat in moderation.

f. Pea Protein Powder: Pea protein is a low-phosphorus, plant-based choice that may be readily added to your smoothies.

3. Hydration-Boosting Ingredients

Staying well-hydrated is vital for kidney health. Smoothies may be an excellent approach to enhance your fluid consumption while integrating hydrating elements. Consider adding these hydration-boosting ingredients to your kidney-friendly smoothies:

a. Coconut Water: Coconut water is a natural electrolyte-rich beverage that increases hydration without additional phosphorus.

b. Watermelon: Watermelon has a high water content and is low in potassium, making it a good option for kidney-friendly hydration.

c. Cilantro: Cilantro not only provides a burst of flavor to your smoothies but also has diuretic effects that encourage fluid balance.

d. Celery: Celery is hydrating and may give a nice, light flavor to your smoothies.

e. Aloe Vera Juice: Aloe vera juice helps ease the digestive tract and enhance hydration, helping kidney function.

f. Green Tea (cooled): Green tea is a hydrating beverage that delivers antioxidants and may be utilized as a liquid foundation for your smoothies.

By carefully choosing these kidney-friendly ingredients, you can produce tasty and nutritious smoothies that are light on the kidneys while giving a broad variety of health advantages. Experiment with various combinations to discover the tastes that best fit your palette and dietary demands. The next chapters will present kidney-friendly smoothie recipes that integrate these healthy components, guaranteeing you may experience the power of smoothies for your kidney health.

# Chapter 5

Supercharged Kidney-Boosting Smoothie Recipes

Smoothies give a terrific chance to fill your diet with kidney-boosting nutrients and pleasant tastes. In this chapter, we will explore six delightful and nutrient-packed smoothie recipes particularly intended to enhance kidney health and general well-being. Each recipe combines a range of kidney-friendly ingredients to give a surge of nutrients, making these smoothies a fantastic addition to your daily routine.

1. Berry Blast Smoothie

Berries are rich in antioxidants, low in potassium, and high in fiber, making them great for kidney health. This Berry Blast Smoothie mixes the richness of several berries to produce a pleasant and nutrient-packed treat.

Ingredients:

1 cup mixed berries (strawberries, blueberries, raspberries)

1/2 banana

1/2 cup unsweetened almond milk

1 tbsp chia seeds

1 tablespoon honey (optional for extra sweetness)

Ice cubes (optional, for a cold smoothie)

2. Green Goddess Detox Smoothie

This Green Goddess Detox Smoothie blends kidney-cleansing components, such as cucumber and cilantro, with nutrient-rich leafy greens, making it a perfect option for detoxing and maintaining kidney function.

Ingredients:

1 cup spinach

1/2 cucumber

1/2 avocado

1/2 cup fresh cilantro leaves

1/2 lemon (juiced)

1 cup coconut water

Ice cubes (optional, for a cold smoothie)

3. Pineapple with Turmeric Elixir

Turmeric has significant anti-inflammatory effects, and paired with pineapple's tropical sweetness, this smoothie provides a tasty method to promote kidney health.

Ingredients:

1 cup pineapple chunks

1/2 teaspoon ground turmeric

1/2 cup Greek yogurt (low-fat or non-fat)

1 tablespoon flaxseed

1/2 cup water or almond milk

1 teaspoon honey (optional, for extra sweetness)

Ice cubes (optional, for a cold smoothie)

4. Creamy Avocado Delight

Avocado delivers healthy fats that improve satiety and aid nutrient absorption, while spinach gives a nutritious boost to this Creamy Avocado Delight smoothie.

Ingredients:

1/2 avocado

1 cup spinach

1/2 cup cucumber

1/2 cup unsweetened coconut milk

1 tablespoon hemp seeds

1/2 teaspoon grated ginger

Ice cubes (optional, for a cold smoothie)

# 5. Citrusy Carrot Cleanser

Citrus fruits are rich in vitamin C and antioxidants, while carrots provide natural sweetness and a plethora of vitamins and minerals to this delightful Citrusy Carrot Cleanser.

Ingredients:

1 orange (peeled and segmented)

1/2 cup carrots (sliced)

1/2 cup coconut water

1 tablespoon fresh lime juice

1 tbsp chia seeds

Ice cubes (optional, for a cold smoothie)

## 6. Antioxidant Powerhouse Smoothie

This Antioxidant Powerhouse Smoothie combines a range of antioxidant-rich foods, including blueberries, kale, and green tea, to promote kidney health and general well-being.

Ingredients:

1 cup blueberries

1 cup kale (stems removed)

1/2 cup brewed green tea (cooled)

1/2 banana

1 tablespoon honey (optional, for extra sweetness)

Ice cubes (optional, for a cold smoothie)

Directions for all smoothies:

Add all the ingredients to a blender.

Blend until smooth and creamy.

Adjust the consistency by adding additional liquid if required.

Pour into a glass and enjoy your supercharged kidney-boosting smoothie!

These kidney-friendly smoothie recipes provide a tasty approach to filling your body with critical nutrients while promoting renal health. Feel free to adapt the recipes according to your taste preferences and nutritional demands. Regularly including these smoothies in your diet may help greatly to better kidney function and general well-being.

# Chapter 6

Smoothies for Specific Kidney Conditions

While smoothies may be a terrific complement to any kidney-friendly diet, personalizing them to suit particular kidney diseases can boost their benefits. In this chapter, we will study four kinds of smoothies intended to treat various kidney conditions: Kidney Stones, Diabetic-Friendly Kidney Smoothies, Hypertension and Renal Health Smoothies, and Dialysis Supportive Smoothie Recipes. Each set of smoothies focuses on certain minerals and ingredients to help manage these diseases and promote improved kidney function.

1. Smoothies for Kidney Stones

Kidney stones may cause extreme pain and agony, and treating them via dietary choices is vital. Smoothies for Kidney Stones should concentrate on elements that improve hydration, minimize the chance of stone development, and calm the urinary system.

Ingredients to Consider:

Citrus Fruits: Lemon, lime, and oranges are strong in citric acid, which may help avoid some forms of kidney stones.

Cucumbers: Cucumbers have high water content and may assist in keeping hydrated.

Watermelon: Watermelon is a hydrating fruit that may improve kidney function and help flush out toxins.

Sample Recipe: Citrus-Cucumber Cooler

- 1/2 cup fresh lemon juice

- 

- 1/2 cup fresh cucumber slices

- 

- 1 cup watermelon chunks

- 

- 1 cup coconut water

- 

- Ice cubes (optional)

## 2. Diabetic-Friendly Kidney Smoothies

For those with diabetes and kidney issues, regulating blood sugar levels is critical.

Diabetic-Friendly Kidney Smoothies should concentrate on low-glycemic components and nutrient-dense meals that help blood sugar management and kidney function.

Ingredients to Consider:

Leafy Greens: Spinach and kale are low in carbohydrates and abundant in nutrients, making them good alternatives for diabetics.

Berries: Berries have a low glycemic index and are rich in antioxidants.

Cinnamon: Cinnamon may assist enhance insulin sensitivity and blood sugar management.

Sample Recipe: Berry-Green Delight

- 1 cup spinach

- 

- 1/2 cup mixed berries (strawberries, blueberries, raspberries)

- 

- 1 tbsp chia seeds

- 1 teaspoon ground cinnamon

- 

- 1/2 cup unsweetened almond milk

- 

- Ice cubes (optional)

Hypertension and Renal Health Smoothies

3. Hypertension (high blood pressure) may lead to kidney damage, thus concentrating on substances that promote cardiovascular health is important. Hypertension and Renal Health Smoothies should contain

foods rich in potassium, calcium, and antioxidants.

Ingredients to Consider:

Kale: Kale is rich in potassium and calcium, both vital for heart and kidney health.

Beets: Beets contain nitrates that may help decrease blood pressure.

Blueberries: Blueberries are filled with antioxidants that aid the cardiovascular system.


Sample Recipe: Heart-Healthy Beet-Berry Blend

- 1 cup kale

-

- 1/2 cup cooked beets (sliced)

-

- 1/2 cup blueberries

-

- 1 tablespoon flaxseed

- 

- 1/2 cup water or unsweetened coconut water

- 

- Ice cubes (optional)

4. Dialysis Supportive Smoothie Recipes

For those on dialysis, it's vital to monitor fluid and nutritional intake. Dialysis Supportive Smoothie Recipes should concentrate on foods that are low in potassium, phosphorus, and salt while boosting hydration.

Ingredients to Consider:

Apple: Apples are low in potassium and phosphorus and may give natural sweetness to smoothies.

Rice Milk: Rice milk is a low-phosphorus milk replacement that may be used as a liquid foundation.

Strawberries: Strawberries are a kidney-friendly fruit with a low potassium concentration.

Sample Recipe: Apple-Strawberry Delight

- 1/2 apple (peeled and diced)

- 

- 1/2 cup strawberries

- 

- 1 cup rice milk

- 

- 1 tablespoon hemp seeds

- 

- 1/2 teaspoon vanilla extract

- 

- Ice cubes (optional)

Remember, persons with certain renal diseases must work closely with their healthcare team, especially a trained dietitian, to adapt their smoothies and dietary choices according to their unique needs and medical requirements. These smoothie recipes may serve as a starting point, offering ideas for making tasty and kidney-friendly drinks that complement a specific renal health plan.

# Chapter 7

Herbal Additions for Enhanced Kidney Health

Nature provides a treasure trove of herbs that can be beneficial for kidney health. In this chapter, we will explore two essential aspects of incorporating herbal additions into your diet for enhanced kidney health: Herbal Teas and Infusions for Kidney Cleansing and Herbal Supplements to Support Kidney Function. These herbal remedies can complement a kidney-friendly lifestyle and offer valuable support to your kidneys' well-being.

1. Herbal Teas and Infusions for Kidney Cleansing

Herbal teas and infusions have been used for centuries to support various aspects of health, including kidney function. The following herbal additions can aid in kidney cleansing and promote a healthy urinary system:

a. Dandelion Root: Dandelion root has diuretic properties that can help flush out excess fluids and toxins from the kidneys and urinary tract.

b. Nettle Leaf: Nettle leaf is known for its detoxifying properties and may help in maintaining kidney health by supporting fluid balance.

c. Corn Silk: Corn silk is a soothing herb that can be brewed into a tea to support the urinary system and promote kidney health.

d. Parsley: Parsley is a popular culinary herb that can also be used as a tea. It is known for its diuretic effects and potential to support kidney function.

e. Hibiscus: Hibiscus tea has been shown to support healthy blood pressure levels, which is beneficial for kidney health.

f. Marshmallow Root: Marshmallow root has a soothing effect on the urinary system and can be used in teas or infusions for kidney support.

## Herbal Tea Recipe: Kidney Cleansing Infusion

- 1 teaspoon dried nettle leaf
- 1 teaspoon dried dandelion root
- 1 teaspoon dried corn silk
- 1 cup boiling water
- Honey or lemon (optional, for added flavor)

Instructions:

1. In a teapot or mug, add the dried nettle leaf, dandelion root, and corn silk.

2. Pour the hot water over the herbs and let it sit for 5-10 minutes.

3. Strain the infusion into another cup.

4. Add honey or lemon, if desired, for added flavor.

5. Enjoy this kidney-cleansing infusion daily as part of your kidney health routine.

2. Herbal Supplements to Support Kidney Function

In addition to herbal teas and infusions, herbal supplements can be beneficial for supporting kidney function and overall kidney health. It's essential to consult with a healthcare professional or a registered herbalist before adding any herbal supplement to your diet, especially if you have existing health conditions or are taking medications. Some herbal supplements that may offer kidney support include:

a. Astragalus: Astragalus is an herb used in traditional Chinese medicine to support kidney health and overall vitality.

b. Milk Thistle: Milk thistle is known for its liver-supportive properties, but it can also have potential benefits for kidney function.

c. Cordyceps: Cordyceps is a medicinal mushroom with potential protective effects on kidney health.

d. Buchu: Buchu is an African herb traditionally used to support urinary health and kidney function.

e. Chanca Piedra: Chanca piedra is a herb commonly used in South America for its potential to support kidney and urinary health.

Important Note: Herbal supplements can interact with medications and may not be suitable for everyone. Always consult with your healthcare provider before starting any new herbal supplements, especially if you are pregnant, nursing, or have underlying health conditions.

Incorporating herbal teas, infusions, and supplements can be a valuable addition to a kidney-friendly diet and lifestyle. These herbal additions offer natural support for kidney health and can complement other dietary and lifestyle modifications. Remember to approach herbal remedies with caution and always seek professional advice to ensure their safety and efficacy for your specific needs.

# Chapter 8

Incorporating Smoothies into a Kidney-Friendly Lifestyle

Integrating kidney-friendly smoothies into your daily routine is just one aspect of maintaining optimal kidney health. In this chapter, we will explore six vital components to consider when incorporating smoothies into a kidney-friendly lifestyle. These elements will help create a balanced and holistic approach to supporting your kidneys and overall well-being.

1. Creating a Balanced Diet Plan

While smoothies are a nutritious addition to your diet, it's essential to incorporate them into a balanced meal plan that supports kidney health. A balanced diet for kidney health should include:

a. Appropriate Portions: Pay attention to portion sizes, especially regarding potassium, phosphorus, sodium, and protein intake, to prevent overburdening the kidneys.

b. Nutrient-Rich Foods: Emphasize fruits, vegetables, whole grains, lean proteins, and healthy fats to provide essential nutrients without overloading the kidneys.

c. Limiting Processed Foods: Reduce the consumption of processed and high-sodium foods, which can contribute to kidney damage and other health issues.

d. Fluid Intake: Adjust your fluid intake according to your specific kidney condition and medical recommendations.

e. Regular Monitoring: Regularly monitor your kidney function and adjust your diet plan accordingly with the guidance of a registered dietitian or healthcare professional.

2. The Role of Exercise in Kidney Health

Physical activity is crucial for kidney health and overall well-being. Regular exercise can help:

a. Manage Blood Pressure: Physical activity can help lower blood pressure, reducing the risk of kidney damage.

b. Control Blood Sugar: Exercise can improve insulin sensitivity, benefiting those with diabetes-related kidney concerns.

c. Promote Weight Management: Maintaining a healthy weight can reduce the strain on the kidneys.

d. Improve Cardiovascular Health: Exercise supports heart health, which is directly linked to kidney function.

e. Enhance Mood and Mental Health: Physical activity can reduce stress and promote emotional well-being.

3. Managing Stress for Optimal Kidney Function

Chronic stress can negatively impact kidney health and exacerbate existing kidney conditions. Implement stress management techniques to support your kidneys, such as:

a. Mindfulness Meditation: Practicing mindfulness meditation can reduce stress and promote relaxation.

b. Yoga: Engaging in gentle yoga can improve flexibility, reduce tension, and aid in stress reduction.

c. Regular Exercise: Physical activity releases endorphins, which can improve mood and reduce stress.

d. Creative Outlets: Pursue creative hobbies or activities that bring joy and serve as a positive outlet for stress.

e. Support Systems: Seek support from friends, family, or support groups to help manage stress and emotional challenges.

4. Quality Sleep for Kidney Health

Adequate sleep is essential for kidney health and overall well-being. It is recommended to get 7-9 hours of good sleep each night. Good sleep habits can:

a. Promote Cellular Repair: During sleep, the body repairs and rejuvenates tissues, including the kidneys.

b. Regulate Hormones: Proper sleep helps regulate hormones that impact kidney function.

c. Enhance Immune Function: Quality sleep supports a robust immune system, protecting against infections that could affect the kidneys.

d. Improve Mood and Mental Health: Lack of sleep can contribute to stress and negatively impact mental health.

e. Support Cardiovascular Health: Sufficient sleep is crucial for heart health, which is closely linked to kidney function.

5. Staying Hydrated and Mindful of Fluid Intake

Proper hydration is vital for kidney health, but individuals with specific kidney conditions may have fluid restrictions. Follow your healthcare provider's guidelines regarding fluid intake. To stay hydrated:

a. Monitor Fluid Intake: Keep track of your daily fluid intake to ensure it aligns with your medical recommendations.

b. Choose Hydrating Foods: Incorporate hydrating foods like fruits and vegetables into your diet.

c. Sip Throughout the Day: Spread your fluid intake throughout the day instead of consuming large amounts all at once.

d. Be Mindful of Beverages: Be aware of the fluid content in beverages, including smoothies, soups, and other liquids.

6. Regular Health Checkups and Monitoring

Regular health checkups and kidney function monitoring are essential for maintaining kidney health. Schedule regular visits with your healthcare provider, especially if you have existing kidney concerns or are at risk for kidney issues. Monitoring kidney function can help identify any changes or potential problems early, allowing for timely intervention and management.

Incorporating kidney-friendly smoothies into your lifestyle goes hand in hand with mindful dietary choices, regular exercise, stress management, quality sleep, hydration, and monitoring your health. This holistic approach empowers you to take charge of your kidney health, supporting your kidneys' well-being and contributing to a happier, healthier life.

# Chapter 9

Tips for a Successful Kidney-Friendly Smoothie Journey

Embarking on a kidney-friendly smoothie journey can be a rewarding experience that supports your kidney health and overall well-being. To ensure a successful and enjoyable journey, consider the following six tips that cover everything from shopping for kidney-friendly ingredients to customizing your smoothies according to personal taste and preferences.

1. Shopping for Kidney-Friendly Ingredients

A successful kidney-friendly smoothie journey begins with selecting the right ingredients. When you hit the stores, remember to keep these things in mind:

a. Read Labels: Check the nutritional content on food labels for potassium, phosphorus, sodium, and protein content to make informed choices.

b. Choose Fresh Produce: Opt for fresh fruits and vegetables when possible, as they tend to have lower sodium and preservative content.

c. Buy Frozen Options: Frozen fruits and vegetables can be just as nutritious as fresh ones and offer convenience without the risk of spoilage.

d.   Low-Potassium   Fruits:   Prioritize low-potassium fruits like berries, apples, and pears to avoid overloading your kidneys.

e. Herbal Additions: Consider incorporating kidney-friendly herbs like parsley or dandelion greens for added health benefits.

2. Batch Prepping and Storage Tips

Efficient batch prepping and storage can make incorporating smoothies into your daily routine much easier:

a. Wash and Prep in Advance: Wash, peel, and chop fruits and vegetables in advance to save time when making smoothies.

b. Freeze in Portions: Pre-measure smoothie ingredients and freeze them in individual portions for quick and easy blending.

c. Use Mason Jars: Prepare smoothie ingredients in mason jars and store them in the refrigerator for a grab-and-go option.

d. Label and Date: Label your frozen smoothie ingredients with the type and date to keep track of freshness.

e. Consider Smoothie Packs: Create pre-made smoothie packs with all the necessary ingredients, so you only need to add liquid and blend.

3. Adjusting Smoothies for Personal Taste and Preference

Customizing your smoothies to suit your taste preferences ensures you'll enjoy your kidney-friendly smoothie journey:

a. Sweetness Level: Adjust the sweetness of your smoothies by using ripe fruits or natural sweeteners like honey or stevia.

b. Texture: Experiment with different ingredients to achieve your desired smoothie texture, whether thick and creamy or light and refreshing.

c. Liquid Base: Try different liquid bases like almond milk, coconut water, or green tea to add unique flavors to your smoothies.

d. Superfoods: Enhance the nutritional profile of your smoothies by adding superfoods like chia seeds, flaxseed, or spirulina.

e. Protein Choices: Switch up your protein sources between plant-based options like hemp seeds or animal-based options like Greek yogurt (if suitable for your dietary needs).

4. Avoid Smoothie Burnout

To prevent smoothie burnout and maintain your enthusiasm for kidney-friendly smoothies:

a. Rotate Ingredients: Regularly switch up your smoothie ingredients to keep the flavors fresh and exciting.

b. Explore New Recipes: Look for new kidney-friendly smoothie recipes online or in books to inspire your taste buds.

c. Set a Schedule: Create a smoothie schedule that incorporates different flavors and themes throughout the week.

d. Share with Others: Share your favorite smoothie recipes with friends and family to encourage a sense of community and support.

e. Be Creative: Don't be afraid to experiment and get creative with your smoothie combinations to keep things interesting.

5 Monitor Nutrient Intake

Keep track of your nutrient intake, especially if you have specific dietary restrictions:

a. Use Apps or Journals: Utilize apps or food journals to monitor your nutrient intake, including potassium, phosphorus, sodium, and protein.

b. Consult with a Dietitian: Work with a registered dietitian who specializes in kidney health to create a personalized dietary plan.

c. Balance Smoothies with Meals: Ensure your smoothies complement your overall diet and do not lead to nutrient imbalances.

6. Celebrate Progress and Stay Consistent

Lastly, celebrate your progress on your kidney-friendly smoothie journey and stay consistent with your healthy habits:

a. Set Goals: Establish achievable goals for your smoothie journey and celebrate your milestones.

b. Establish Routine: Incorporate smoothies into your daily routine for consistent kidney support.

c. Seek Support: Connect with others who are on a similar journey to share experiences and advice.

d. Listen to Your Body: Pay attention to how your body responds to the changes and adjust as needed.

e. Be Patient: Improving kidney health takes time, so be patient with yourself and stay committed to your well-being.

By following these tips, you'll embark on a successful kidney-friendly smoothie journey that enhances your kidney health, supports overall wellness, and makes nourishing choices a delightful part of your daily life.

# Chapter 10

Precautions and Considerations

While incorporating kidney-friendly smoothies into your lifestyle can be beneficial, it's essential to approach this journey with caution and mindfulness. This chapter covers three critical considerations to ensure a safe and effective experience with kidney-friendly smoothies: Consulting with a Healthcare Professional, Potential Interactions with Medications, and Monitoring Progress and Adjusting Smoothie Plans.

1. Consulting with a Healthcare Professional

Before making significant changes to your diet, especially if you have existing kidney issues or medical conditions, consult with a healthcare professional, such as a nephrologist or a registered dietitian. They can provide personalized guidance based on your specific health needs, kidney function, and medical history. A healthcare professional can help you create a kidney-friendly meal plan, including smoothies, that aligns with your dietary restrictions, nutrient requirements, and overall health goals.

2. Potential Interactions with Medications

Some ingredients commonly used in smoothies, including herbs and supplements, may interact with certain medications. Herbal supplements, in particular, can have potent effects and may interfere with medications used to manage kidney conditions or other health issues. Inform your healthcare provider about any herbal additions you plan to incorporate into your smoothies to ensure there are no adverse interactions with your medications. Your healthcare provider can also recommend kidney-safe supplements, if necessary.

3. Monitoring Progress and Adjusting Smoothie Plans

As you introduce kidney-friendly smoothies into your diet, it's essential to monitor your progress and adapt your smoothie plans as needed. Pay attention to the following:

a. Kidney Function: If you have kidney issues, continue to monitor your kidney function through regular checkups and lab tests.

b. Fluid Intake: If you are on fluid restrictions, keep track of your fluid intake, including smoothies, to ensure compliance with your prescribed limits.

c. Nutrient Levels: Monitor your intake of key nutrients, such as potassium, phosphorus, sodium, and protein, to avoid overloading your kidneys.

d. Allergies and Sensitivities: Be mindful of any allergies or sensitivities to ingredients in your smoothies and make adjustments accordingly.

e. Personal Tolerance: Listen to your body and make modifications to your smoothie recipes if certain ingredients cause discomfort or adverse reactions.

Remember that every individual's health needs are unique, and what works well for one person may not be suitable for another. Being attentive to your body's responses and regularly communicating with your healthcare team will help you tailor your smoothie journey to best support your kidney health and overall well-being.

In conclusion, while kidney-friendly smoothies can be a valuable addition to a kidney-friendly lifestyle, taking precautions and seeking professional guidance is essential to ensure a safe and effective experience. By consulting with healthcare professionals, being aware of potential medication interactions, and regularly monitoring your progress, you can confidently enjoy the benefits of kidney-friendly smoothies while safeguarding your health. Embrace this journey with care, and you'll discover how nourishing and supporting your kidneys can lead to improved overall wellness and vitality.

# Chapter 11

Frequently Asked Questions about Kidney Health and Smoothies - Addressing Common Concerns and Misconceptions

As the popularity of kidney-friendly smoothies grows, so do the questions and concerns surrounding their suitability for kidney health. In this chapter, we will address some of the most common concerns and misconceptions related to kidney health and smoothies. By clarifying these issues, we aim to provide you with a better understanding of how smoothies can be incorporated into a kidney-friendly lifestyle.

Q1: Can smoothies worsen kidney function due to their potassium content?

A1: Smoothies can be a source of potassium, especially if they contain potassium-rich fruits and vegetables like bananas or oranges. However, with proper portion control and attention to ingredients, smoothies can be part of a balanced diet that supports kidney health. Opt for lower-potassium fruits like berries and apples, and work with a registered dietitian to determine appropriate portion sizes based on your specific kidney function.

Q2: Are green smoothies safe for kidney health?

A2: Green smoothies made with kidney-friendly ingredients like leafy greens and low-potassium fruits can be safe and beneficial for kidney health. Leafy greens like spinach and kale provide essential nutrients without overloading the kidneys with potassium. Be mindful of the total potassium content in your smoothies and avoid high-potassium greens like Swiss chard or beet greens.

Q3: Do smoothies contribute to kidney stones?

A3: Smoothies made with ingredients like citrus fruits and cucumber, which can have a kidney stone-preventing effect, may actually reduce the risk of kidney stone formation. However, it's essential to maintain a balanced diet and moderate your intake of high-oxalate ingredients like spinach and beets, as excessive oxalates can contribute to certain types of kidney stones.

Q4: Can smoothies lead to excessive fluid intake for those on fluid restrictions?

A4: For individuals on fluid restrictions, it's crucial to monitor their overall fluid intake, including the liquids in smoothies. You can control the fluid content of your smoothies by adjusting the amount of liquid used or opting for ingredients with lower water content. Work with your healthcare team to determine an appropriate fluid allowance and incorporate smoothies accordingly.

Q5: Can protein-rich smoothies be harmful to the kidneys?

A5: While protein is essential for overall health, excessive protein intake can place a strain on the kidneys. For individuals with kidney issues, it's crucial to balance protein intake and consider low-phosphorus protein sources like chia seeds, hemp seeds, or egg whites. Protein portions in smoothies should align with your dietary needs and medical recommendations.

Q6: Are herbal additions in smoothies safe for kidney health?

A6: Herbal additions like dandelion root or nettle leaf may have potential benefits for kidney health, but they should be used with caution. Some herbs can interact with medications or have diuretic effects, impacting fluid balance. Consult with a healthcare professional before adding herbal additions to your smoothies, especially if you have existing kidney issues or are taking medications.

Q7: Can smoothies replace medications for kidney conditions?

A7: Smoothies are not a substitute for prescribed medications or medical treatments for kidney conditions. While they can support kidney health, they should be part of a comprehensive approach that includes proper medical care, a balanced diet, regular exercise, and lifestyle modifications. Always follow your healthcare provider's recommendations for managing kidney conditions.

Q8: Can I enjoy smoothies if I have diabetes and kidney issues?

A8: Individuals with diabetes and kidney issues can incorporate kidney-friendly smoothies into their diet with proper adjustments. Focus on low-glycemic fruits, monitor sugar content, and consider adding ingredients like cinnamon or avocados to enhance the nutritional profile and manage blood sugar levels. Consult with a registered dietitian to create customized smoothie plans that align with your health needs.

By addressing these common concerns and misconceptions, we hope to empower you with accurate information and guidance on how to embrace kidney-friendly smoothies as a positive addition to your health journey. Remember that personalized nutrition advice from a registered dietitian and regular communication with your healthcare team are essential for making informed decisions that support your kidney health and overall well-being.

# Chapter 12

Success Stories and Testimonials - Real-Life Accounts of People Benefiting from Kidney-Friendly Smoothies

In this chapter, we share inspiring success stories and testimonials from individuals who have experienced the positive impact of incorporating kidney-friendly smoothies into their lives. These personal accounts highlight how smoothies have played a significant role in supporting kidney health and overall well-being.

Testimonial 1: Jessica's Journey to Improved Kidney Function

Jessica, 45, was diagnosed with chronic kidney disease (CKD) and was struggling to manage her condition effectively. Concerned about the impact of her diet on her kidneys, Jessica decided to explore kidney-friendly alternatives. After consulting with a registered dietitian, she started incorporating nutrient-dense smoothies into her daily routine.

"I was extremely shocked when I began drinking kidney-friendly smoothies and noticed the fantastic effects. Not only did my energy levels increase, but my kidney function also improved. I focused on low-potassium fruits, like berries and apples, and included kidney-cleansing ingredients like cucumber and lemon. I feel more in control of my health, and smoothies have become a delicious way to nourish my body and support my kidneys."

Testimonial 2: Mark's Journey to Kidney Health Maintenance

Mark, 62, was managing hypertension and kidney issues for several years. He struggled to find ways to incorporate kidney-friendly foods into his diet. With the guidance of his healthcare team, he discovered the benefits of smoothies for kidney health.

"Smoothies have been a game-changer for me. They've allowed me to incorporate a variety of kidney-friendly ingredients that I wouldn't have considered otherwise. I love using almond milk as a base and adding spinach and berries for added nutrition. Not only have my blood pressure and kidney function stabilized, but I also find joy in experimenting with new smoothie recipes. They've become an essential part of my daily routine, and I'm grateful for the positive impact they've had on my health."

Testimonial 3: Sarah's Kidney-Friendly Smoothie Journey

Sarah, 29, had kidney stones and was determined to take proactive steps to prevent them from recurring. She started exploring kidney-friendly smoothies as a way to support her urinary health.

"I was prepared to do whatever it took to avoid suffering through kidney stones again because I was determined to avoid the pain and exhaustion they cause.

Smoothies became a fun and tasty way for me to hydrate and support my kidneys. I focused on citrus fruits like lemons and oranges, which are known for their kidney stone-preventing properties. I also added cucumbers and watermelon to stay hydrated. Since incorporating smoothies into my diet, I haven't had any kidney stone episodes, and I feel more confident about my kidney health."

Testimonial 4: John's Journey to a Refreshing Kidney-Friendly Diet

John, 55, was struggling with fluid restrictions due to kidney issues. He found it challenging to stay hydrated while adhering to his prescribed fluid limit. Kidney-friendly smoothies became a creative solution.

"I used to absolutely despise being limited on fluids since I was always so darn thirsty. But then I discovered smoothies as a way to enjoy delicious and hydrating beverages within my limits. I prepared pre-portioned smoothie packs with low-potassium fruits, like blueberries and peaches, and blended them with coconut water. Not only did it help me stay hydrated, but it also made drinking fluids more enjoyable. Smoothies have become a refreshing part of my daily routine, and I no longer feel restricted by my fluid intake."

These success stories and testimonials exemplify the positive impact of kidney-friendly smoothies on real people's lives. Each individual found their unique way to incorporate smoothies into their diets, and the results were both beneficial and motivating. As you continue on your own kidney-friendly smoothie journey, remember that these accounts are an encouragement to explore the countless possibilities smoothies offer for supporting kidney health and overall well-being. Always consult with your healthcare team to create a personalized plan that aligns with your health needs and enjoy the journey of nourishing your body and kidneys through flavorful and nutritious smoothies.

# Conclusion

Embracing a Kidney-Healthy Lifestyle with Smoothies

Congratulations on completing this journey through "Smoothies for Kidney Health"! As you've learned, kidney-friendly smoothies can be a powerful tool for supporting kidney health and overall well-being. By incorporating nutrient-dense and delicious smoothies into your daily routine, you've taken a proactive step toward enhancing your kidney health and embracing a more balanced lifestyle.

Throughout this book, we've explored the importance of understanding kidney function, common kidney health issues, and the role of diet and exercise in supporting kidney well-being. We've delved into the power of smoothies and their benefits for kidneys, and you've discovered a wide array of kidney-friendly ingredients to create delicious and nourishing smoothie recipes.

The journey doesn't end here! As you continue your kidney-healthy lifestyle with smoothies, keep these key takeaways in mind:

- Personalization is Key: Every person's health needs are unique, and it's essential to tailor your smoothie plans to align with your specific kidney function, medical recommendations, and taste preferences. Consulting with a healthcare professional and a registered dietitian can help you create a customized plan that supports your health journey.

- Quality Ingredients Matter: Choose high-quality, kidney-friendly ingredients for your smoothies. Emphasize low-potassium fruits, non-starchy vegetables, and low-phosphorus proteins to nourish your body and kidneys while avoiding overloading them with certain nutrients.

- Balance and Moderation: Balance is the cornerstone of a kidney-healthy lifestyle. Moderation is key when it comes to nutrients like potassium, phosphorus, sodium, protein, and fluids. Pay attention to portion sizes and nutrient content to maintain a balanced diet.

- Regular Monitoring: Keep track of your kidney function, fluid intake, and nutrient levels through regular checkups and lab tests. Monitoring progress and staying proactive can help you make informed adjustments to your kidney-friendly smoothie plans.

- Wellness Beyond Smoothies: Kidney-friendly smoothies are just one aspect of a holistic approach to kidney health. Engage in regular exercise, manage stress, get quality sleep, and maintain open communication with your healthcare team to support your kidneys and overall well-being.

Remember that embracing a kidney-healthy lifestyle with smoothies is not about restriction or sacrifice. It's about nurturing your body with nourishing and delicious ingredients that promote kidney health and overall vitality. Enjoy the journey of creating new smoothie recipes, experimenting with flavors, and finding what works best for you.

As you venture forth, we encourage you to share your own success stories and experiences with kidney-friendly smoothies. Your journey may inspire others to take charge of their kidney health and embark on their own path to wellness.

Thank you for joining us on this enriching and healthful journey. We wish you a vibrant and kidney-healthy life filled with the joy of savoring each kidney-friendly smoothie you create. Cheers to your health and well-being!

# Bonus Chapter

Kidney-Friendly Smoothie Ingredients

Kidney-friendly smoothies are a delightful and nutritious way to support kidney health and overall well-being. When creating these smoothies, it's essential to choose ingredients that are low in potassium, phosphorus, and sodium, while also providing essential nutrients and hydration. Below are some kidney-friendly smoothie ingredients to consider incorporating into your recipes:

1. Low-Potassium Fruits: Opt for fruits with lower potassium content to avoid burdening the kidneys. Some excellent choices include

blueberries, strawberries, raspberries, apples, pears, peaches, and watermelon.

2. Non-Starchy Vegetables: Vegetables are packed with vitamins and minerals while being lower in potassium and phosphorus. Consider adding spinach, kale, cucumber, zucchini, and celery to your smoothies.

3. Low-Phosphorus Proteins: Choose protein sources that are lower in phosphorus to support kidney health. Some options include hemp seeds, chia seeds, flaxseed, egg whites, and unsweetened almond or rice milk.

4. Hydration-Boosting Ingredients: Staying hydrated is vital for kidney health.

Incorporate hydrating ingredients like coconut water, watermelon, and cucumber into your smoothies.

5. Citrus Fruits: Citrus fruits like lemons and limes are excellent additions to kidney-friendly smoothies. They are refreshing, hydrating, and can help prevent kidney stones.

6. Avocado: Avocado adds creaminess and healthy fats to smoothies without being too high in potassium.

7. Cinnamon: Cinnamon can add a delightful flavor to smoothies without contributing to potassium or phosphorus levels.

8. Greek Yogurt (in moderation): If your diet allows for some dairy, consider using small amounts of low-phosphorus Greek yogurt for added creaminess and protein.

9. Herbal Additions: Some herbs, like parsley and dandelion greens, may have kidney-cleansing properties and can be added to smoothies in moderation.

10. Ice Cubes or Frozen Ingredients: Using ice cubes or frozen fruits and vegetables can create a refreshing and cool smoothie while reducing the need for added liquid.

Remember that the key to kidney-friendly smoothies is balance and moderation. Be mindful of portion sizes and nutrient content to support your kidney health. Additionally, individual dietary needs may vary, so it's essential to consult with a healthcare professional or a registered dietitian to create personalized smoothie recipes that align with your specific health goals and medical recommendations. Enjoy the process of creating delicious and nourishing kidney-friendly smoothies, and savor the benefits they bring to your well-being!

Note: Before making significant changes to one's diet, especially for individuals with existing health conditions, it's crucial to consult with a healthcare professional or a registered dietitian to ensure the smoothie recipes align with their specific needs and health status. This book aims to provide helpful information and recipes but should not replace personalized medical advice.